NO CHILDREN,
NO GUILT

Sylvia D. Lucas

For you.

CONTENTS

Acknowledgements   i

1   How Could Anyone *Not* Want Children?   4

2   Accept Your Disinclination Toward Motherhood   16

3   Telling People   28

4   Dealing with the Opposition   40

5   Finding a Mate   46

6   Making It Happen   60

7   Social Awkwardness   69

8   They're Not Judging Just You   79

9   Don't Fear the Question   85

10   Ten Key Points to Remember   96

ACKNOWLEDGMENTS

I'd like to thank the many child-free men and women in the world for trusting their instincts and themselves.

Parenthood isn't for everyone.

INTRODUCTION

Like most women, I've known since I was old enough to think about such things that there was some expectation that because I was female, I would have children. (Woman=Mother.) It wasn't a conscious awareness. That is, I didn't actually think, "They want me to have children." It was just a feeling, a lingering discomfort that somewhere out there, waiting in the mist of the future, were my potential offspring.

My parents didn't communicate any hopeful expectations regarding children; they just made, and expressed, a fairly natural assumption. After I was grounded or lectured or told to do something I thought was completely arbitrary or unreasonable, they would say, "Wait until you have kids of your own. You'll see." Invariably, my first thought would be, "Kids?! What?" The possibility was so far removed from what I envisioned myself doing at any point in my life that I was usually too shocked by the suggestion to reply. But by the time I reached seventeen, I'd had a sexual relationship, and I had been forced more than once to imagine what it would be like to learn I was pregnant. And I could finally say (with confident teenage omniscience) to my parents' accusation that I would do exactly as they were doing when I had children of my own, "I'm never having kids."

Sardonic parental laughter. Snort. "Yes, you are."

The frustration caused by that kind of certainty—that they knew me better than I knew myself—followed me into my twenties, where still more people would assure me I was wrong, that I would change my mind, but in my twenties, a new emotion joined in: guilt. My husbands (I had them one at a time) were fairly traditional, down-home men who didn't necessarily think about having children, but who—like many—simply assumed children would be part of their life course: grow up, get married, have children. When I married my first husband, I was very young, and in the early-stage romantic relationship days of unicorns and rainbows, I thought I *might* be able to want children. In fact, at least once, I couldn't imagine anything better than being in lovey-love and raising heart-shaped babies with him. But as we grew into our relationship and the endorphins settled down, the idea of having children once again felt unnatural. And because I was the only one I knew who didn't want children, I started wondering if it was *I* who was unnatural. If I was *wrong* to not want children. I wondered what people would think of me if they knew, if I said it out loud.

Guilt was later followed by self-worth issues ("You mean, you only want to be with me if I'll have your baby? You don't love me just for me?"), and self-worth issues were followed, with husband number two, by anger ("*Why* would you assume I would change my mind about children? I explicitly told you, 'I don't want children.'").

What is condensed in this introduction to a paragraph and a half spanned approximately thirteen years of real life. Granted, there are those who are immediately comfortable with, and confident about, their decision to not have children. They don't fear telling people, when asked, that they don't ever plan to have a baby, and they're not infuriated when a well-meaning friend says, "Oh, you'll want them some day. Don't worry!" But not everyone is this fortunate. For many, those years spent feeling the pressure of other people's expectations and second-guessing themselves ("*Everyone* wants kids. That has to mean *I* should want them right? Why don't I want them?") can feel like a constant weight. Even if it's not a conscious concern, it's there. But it shouldn't be. It should be as simple as this: If you want children, you want children. If you don't, you don't. Period.

I finally learned the "period" part soon after I turned thirty, and it's my sincere hope that *No Children, No Guilt* will help alleviate any baby-pressure you feel and convince you once and for all that *there is nothing wrong with not wanting children.* (In fact, not having them is a hell of a lot of fun.) - Sylvia

ONE

HOW COULD ANYONE *NOT* WANT CHILDREN?

"Childless-by-choice (aka, "childfree") women literally choose not to have children, either because they flat-out dislike them or because of idealistic religious or environmental reasons."

—Library Journal Review of *The Childless Revolution: What it Means to be Childless Today* by Madelyn Cain

"[...] *because they flat-out dislike them or because of idealistic religious or environmental reasons.*"

Or, for much simpler reasons.

No one tugs at my pants. No one interrupts my shower. No one asks for my already spent energy, or helps deplete the household income.

Spontaneous and uninterrupted sex isn't a "someday" fantasy, and evenings out can last until morning — without a babysitter. Silence, alone time, and free time are all mine, and mornings mean coffee,

4

news, and time to wake up instead of getting into immediate action waking others, making sure they bathe, getting lunches ready, and making sure a permission slip or progress report is signed.

At night, there's nothing to do after work but flop on a soft couch with a remote control and a bowl of soup that's ready to eat after forty-five seconds in the microwave.

It's hard to beat.

Lest I sound callous, I want to share that I have a very vivid memory of my first experience with what I thought at the time wasn't possible: adults not automatically adoring children. It was actually painful when it happened (that is, it sort of hurt my little-girl feelings), but I understand, now.

I was four years old, maybe five, at the time. I'd just been treated rudely by a man who lived in our apartment building. I walked into the small apartment unit we lived in, found my father in the kitchen, and told him about "that" man down the hall.

"I think he just doesn't like kids," my dad said.

I tried to make sense of it. *An adult who didn't like children?*

"How can he not like them?" I said. "He used to be one."

"I don't know," my dad said.

An adult now, I understand that some people simply don't like kids. I also understand that having once been one doesn't mean there's an automatic attraction to them. After all, by the time we reach adulthood, it's as if our child-selves were completely different organisms, and memories of young childhood are less like memories and more like watching someone else's home movies.

But not liking children isn't necessarily the predominant factor contributing to the lack of desire to have one's own children, even if it probably does influence some decisions. Neither, I'm willing to bet, is concern for the environment one of the primary reasons so many women choose not to have children.

These reasons ... the environment, overpopulation, the current state of the world ... are undoubtedly genuine reasons for *some*. But more often, those reasons sound a bit disingenuous, like excuses used by those who feel guilty about simply not wanting children and who feel pressured to provide a good, solid reason others would be hesitant to criticize (face to face, anyway).

There are people, yes, who cannot in any way comprehend that someone might, for no real reason at all, simply not want to have children, and those people are hell-bent on unearthing the *why* behind women not wanting children. *There must be something wrong* (such as a dislike for children, which is not at all acceptable, because women, with their breasts for feeding and their uterus for storing, simply *must* love children) *or something very important in the woman's belief structure* (such as a passion for environmental friendliness) *turning a woman against motherhood*. If the *why* weren't such a fascination, there wouldn't be so many books with titles like, *Unwomanly Conduct: The Challenges of Intentional Childlessness*, by Carolyn M. Morell; *Voluntary Childlessness: The Emergence of a Variant Lifestyle*, by Ellen Mara Nason; and *Without Child: Challenging the Stigma of Childlessness*, by Laurie Lisle.

These titles suggest there is a lot to explore, things to study, stuff to figure out about these mysterious, shady women who don't want children, but conversations with "childfree" women — a preferable term to "childless" by many —hint at a much less interesting reason for the life choice:

We're just not that into it.

Joan C. Chrisler, who has published several books on women's psychology and is the Psychology Department chairwoman at Connecticut College as well as an American Psychological Association and Association for Psychological Science fellow, offered a possible explanation for the driven efforts to explain or analyze voluntary childlessness: "There's the assumption that there must be something wrong with you if you don't want children, because that is supposed to be women's ultimate fulfillment," she said. "There is a pressure in our culture for women to have children. I think all women know that it exists. As soon as heterosexual women get married, people start asking them when they're going to have children. Strangers ask."

- - -

Pregnancy

Childbirth

Crying (mother and baby both)

Potty-training

PTA meetings

Women who don't want children see that list and a strange noise comes from them that sounds a little like "Nn-guh-yuck."

My friend D, who has two brilliant, beautiful children, assures me that even parents who have been looking forward to children since they were children, themselves, don't look forward to any of those things. But the difference, I believe, is that women who want to be parents look at that list and think of it as the unavoidable string of chores that come with raising a child. A necessary evil, I suppose. To them, it's more than worth it. They think (and it's true for them), "But it's all part of the joy of motherhood."

To us, it isn't. That list, to us, is probably best described as the opposite of a bucket list. It's "Things I Really Don't Want to Experience Before I Die—No, Really." And it's not just that we get to avoid the things on that list that makes not having children appealing to those of us who don't want them. There's more. A lot more.

Like, there's a whole lot to love about coming home to a place inhabited only by adults.

Everything is (usually) where it goes, or, at the very least, where you left it. Sharp objects (like figurines with pointy bits or even picture frames) can sit on low shelves, and outlets are exposed for easy plugging and un-plugging. Stairs aren't a hazard to anyone but a drunk.

D said recently, "My friend's daughter spilled eraser fluid on my oak desk."

I don't know what eraser fluid is, but the point is that we childfree don't have to worry about that, either. Will our friends' children ever come over? Maybe—but what are the chances we'll have many friends with children? Slim! (More on that later.)

If we want to go somewhere, we — The Child-free — can pick up and go, whether the destination is a beach six hours away or the drug store down the block. There are no diaper bags to stuff, no children to dress, no wriggling bodies to secure into car seats. Just a walk through the door, a key in the lock, and we're gone.

Even years (and years and years) after moving out of my parents' house, a small thrill continues to accompany the freedom of coming and going without restriction, when I remember to think about it. I don't go out often at night, anymore — I had my extended phase of sneaking out, sneaking in, drinking here and there and back again between the ages of none-of-your-business and none-of-your-business—but if I wanted to, I could. Why, I could stay out until four in the morning. I may not ever do it, but I have the *option*, and that's what matters.

Of course, freedom isn't limited to going out and acting like I'm twenty-one; it's also about greater mobility. Since turning eighteen, I've lived overseas, out East, somewhat West, and sort of South. I could move again tomorrow and the only hassle would be the actual moving part of the move. People with children make frequent moves, too, yes, but moving without children means spending a lot less time on strategizing and fretting. No school districts to choose from, no bus route to worry about, no neighborhood child-predators to look for, no wondering whether there's a playground nearby, and no concerns over whether there are other children close by that my child/ren will get to play with.

When we lived in New York (the state, not the city), my husband and I moved out of our suburban house in a family-friendly (it was an accident) community to a small apartment half a block from what was considered a major downtown street. We were fortunate to be close to one bar with good pizza, another bar with exceptional buffalo wings, a convenience store, and a video store (this was back when video stores were still in business). The only drawback was that someone was killed almost nightly in our city—no exaggeration—and often, it seemed to happen in front of one of those bars.

We even had our very own drug-delivery man. Or, we could have if we'd wanted one. New neighbors who'd moved into the only other unit on our floor (four to the building, two up and two down) 'introduced' us to the dealer. He wasn't a very friendly-looking guy. Maybe if he were it wouldn't have mattered so much. Maybe if he'd smiled, said, "Hi!" and nodded. Something. (No matter the business, one should strive to be friendly and professional.)

The first time my husband and I saw him, we were out on the stoop talking to our downstairs neighbor, R (who claimed to be rap artist Jay-Z's cousin) about where we might be moving next.

Dealer pulled up in a long white car and sat at the curb before honking his horn.

R, a big, tall man, turned to look at Dealer, and then went back to talking to us. The car sat there with the engine running. After a minute or so, R twisted slowly around and said to the elbow poking out of the rolled-down window, "Can I help you?"

"Naw. I'm all right," Dealer said. "Don't worry about it."

R put on his neighborhood voice, shifted his stance. "I ain't worried. You're parked on the street in front of my house. Maybe I can help you out. Maybe they didn't hear your horn."

"They know I'm here," Dealer said.

R turned to us, put his smile back on, once again the friendly-neighbor-let's-grill guy.

"Ain't no reason for you to get scared, or nothin'," Dealer said from his driver's seat.

R stopped smiling. He turned to him. "What was that?"

"I said there ain't no reason for you to be scared."

"Oh," R shook his head, slow-like. "I ain't scared of you."

My husband and I looked at our feet.

I sipped my wine.

He flicked his cigarette.

We tried to look normal, but the way we were looking everywhere but at Dealer or R made it clear we were trying to look normal. One of us may even have whistled.

Certainly, we were happy R stood between us and Dealer's narrow face, narrow eyes, and tight, narrow mouth.

The two talked back and forth, posture this and posture that, before my new neighbor, forty-something with long, dyed-blonde hair and wearing pleated stone-washed jeans, came outside and ran to the car window. She leaned inside, her fuzz-dry hair falling over her shoulders, stuck in her hand, then stepped away and rushed back up the stairs between us. The main door slammed behind her, and Dealer pulled away from the curb in no real hurry.

"You see that?" R said.

We shook our heads. *No way, nu-uh.*

"She just bought some drugs. Came down with a wad of money in her hand. You didn't see that money?"

Me: "M-m."

Husband: "Nope."

R, whose children visited regularly, said, "I don't care if people doin' drugs. My friends come over and get high on my porch, but I don't do none o' that. Like I said,

I don't care if they do it, but don't be sellin' it outside my house."

Husband and I weren't too comfortable with a mean-looking drug dealer pulling up outside of our building, either. What if the couple, living next door and on our floor, their bedroom window next to ours, didn't pay up, one day, and Dealer drove by shooting at the upper floors?

What happened to the good old days when people went to their dealers for the drugs, anyway? I asked R.

R said, "Dealers need the money, now. They got to make housecalls if they want to sell it. Market's dried up."

I'd heard that, too, from R's friends when they were barbequing on his porch a month earlier. I'd opened my kitchen windows for some fresh summer air, and instead caught a whiff of a cloud of happy smoke. When I looked down, I saw a couple of sets of hands stuffing dried, green plant life into rolling papers. There was some talk of drugs, about how they weren't so easy to come by, these days.

"There's a weed shortage," one of them said.

With that kind of activity — people being shot and stabbed, dealers coming to our building — surrounding us, if Husband and I had had children, we'd have had to move. No question. As I understand it, you tend to worry a lot more about your children than you worry about yourselves. But because it was just the two of us we had to look out for, we felt all right about staying until our jobs took us elsewhere. Which meant we were able to squeeze in a few more months of good wings and pizza.

TWO

ACCEPT YOUR DISINCLINATION TOWARD MOTHERHOOD

I can't remember exactly when my initial doubts about motherhood began. My first clue, however, should have come when I was about eight years old and playing in a cave-fort I'd made under the dining room table. Blankets hung over the sides, and doll-daughter and I sat in the dark to wait through an imaginary snowstorm. At some point during that made-up catastrophe, made-up daughter and I had an argument. I threw her on the floor. Then I picked her up and whapped her on the side of the head. I can still see her long red hair whipping around her face.

I'd carry her — and sometimes swing her — by that hair. My dad said once, "How would you like to be carried around like that?"

After I cut her hair into inch-long clumps, I didn't carry her around so much, anymore.

As a little girl, I preferred my toy cars, my machine gun squirt gun, and "spy" glasses to baby dolls and Barbies, and later, as a teen, I noticed there was still a significant difference between the other girls and me. Nothing I can put a finger on even now, but if I had to guess without the benefit of any scientific evidence whatsoever, I would say they simply had more estrogen. They liked painting their nails, reading Sylvia Plath, and carrying Benetton bags. They also seemed to hang out in groups and had bigger breasts than I did.

It *had* to be estrogen.

-

Maybe you were as young as eight when you first suspected you were different, too.

Maybe your friends, eerily adept at such things, would swaddle their dolls in pastel baby blankets, doll-feet tucked inside miniature socks made to look like bunnies or puppy-faces. You, though — you would carry your "baby" around by its barely curled fingers, not noticing when its head smacked doorframes and table corners. You could never quite get the hang of swaddling, always leaving a foot or a hand poking out and exposed to the elements. After trying once or twice to get it right, maybe you ripped off the blanket and tossed it on a pile of Legos in the corner.

Your friends, at doll feeding time, would use a steady hand to wipe imaginary blended peas and carrots from their babies' chins, arranging bibs over tiny torsos while you, fist tight, scraped your doll's face with the spoon and jammed imaginary spit-out peas against its hard, puckered lips, swatting its resin head when you imagined it crying.

After lunch, when it was time to take the babies to the playground, maybe your doll, not even dressed, would dangle at your side like a lunchbox or a worn stuffed animal, bouncing off the pavement when, excited about climbing the wooden ladder to the top of the slide fort, you forgot you were even holding it and let it fall. And as your friends nudged their dolls down the slide or pushed them back and forth, back and forth on the swing, your doll was lost, left behind somewhere in a shaded pit of sand while you took your post in the fort's only tower, swinging an invisible sword at knights from a rival kingdom.

Or maybe you were a teen when it happened. When you were the only one not squeaking at the cuteness of the baby clothes you and your friends passed on the way to the shoe corner.

Your friend Jenny, eyelashes mascara-thick, would pluck a kitten-patterned onesie from the rack and rub the soft cotton between her fingers. "I can't wait to have a baby!" she would say. She was probably bouncing on her toes, smiling wide, smelling the cotton and imagining baby powder.

You, on the other hand, after spotting a mother trying to shush her wailing toddler over by the baby shoes, would think, *Egh*.

You'd look around to make sure no one heard you, that you didn't think it out loud. You'd even smile, maybe say, "Mm!" and finger a pink dress hanging in front of you to show you, too, couldn't wait to play dress-up with a kid.

You began to wonder if you were even supposed to have been born a girl.

It wasn't that you felt like a boy, necessarily. You didn't think you should have a penis, didn't want to grow a beard. But if you weren't dreaming of having a family and an SUV or minivan like all the other girls, what must that mean?

What must that mean?

The mall wasn't the place to think about it, so you waited for your friends to pick and poke their way through the tiny clothes while you, staring somewhere over the perfume counters and thinking about hamburgers, would take a pair of miniature jeans from a rack, absently play with the cuffs, and hang them back up.

Pick up small pair of corduroys.

Smile nurturingly.

Return to rack.

Repeat.

When you were in your twenties, friends bought condoms to avoid catching diseases, and you bought them to avoid catching pregnant first, a disease second.

Once your friends started having babies, houses replaced their apartments, baby-bumpers outfitted furniture corners, and zippy-quick cars were traded in for SUVs to accommodate the one baby, which — with its baby seat, baby bag, baby toys, and baby self — must, you reasoned, need more space than the average car can handle.

(You, not having a baby, would never quite come to understand why something so small couldn't fit in the back seat of a sedan, its accessories in the trunk. Until someone you know would tell you they have the SUV because it's actually safer than a sedan. You would then be tempted to cite studies showing SUVs aren't as safe as advertised, and your friend would argue they're much better for hitting deer. You would, at that point, give up, but you would come to suspect some people use their children as an excuse to buy the SUV they've wanted for years.)

Your apartment, when you were in your twenties, was naturally not baby friendly, and when friends brought their babies over, you would find yourself taking from toddler-hands sparkling geodes, delicate vases, and coasters with sharp edges. Everything you owned, it would seem, was a choking hazard or a cranial danger.

Your friend, sitting cross-legged on the floor and bouncing her baby on its chubby feet, would smile and "goo" and "gah" and press her nose to her child's. Baby fists would curl around Mom's fingers and a shining line of pristine drool would drip like syrup to the floor.

You, watching from the couch with cheeks aching from maintaining the "isn't it cute" smile, would stifle a yawn and wonder why, *why*, you didn't want to bounce that baby, yourself, and why all you could think about was that your friend had only been there ten minutes, and that those ten minutes of keeping things from the baby while making "so cute" noises had you wanting to get drunk and take a bath, and you'd only been out of bed for three hours.

Work wasn't safe, either.

Inevitably, someone would step off the elevator toting a handled baby-seat, newborn swaddled just like the dolls your friends masterfully tucked in those unimaginably soft cotton blankets. You wouldn't even really notice until the sudden "Ohhhh" chorus drifted through the cubicles, and dresses trailing perfume rushed by, stopping short in a cluster by the desk that hadn't been occupied for some odd number of months (you weren't really keeping track) because the woman stationed at that desk had been away on maternity leave.

Maybe you would eye the group of women and wonder if their giggles and enthusiasm were contagious, if maybe you just hadn't given babies enough of a chance.

You would push your chair out from your desk and wander over to the baby-viewing mosh-pit and wait while being nudged back, and back, as women more aggressively interested than you pushed through to get a look, just one look, at that "sweet," "precious," "adorable" face and to have a finger held in the fist everyone would say was uncommonly strong, notably healthy.

Finally, the crowd in front of you would thin enough for you to see the baby if you stood on your toes and looked over the shoulders and through the hair of the women in front of you.

And there it would be.

Yep. A baby, all right.

White socks barely clinging to wrinkled feet, fingers clenching and unclenching, and puffy lips sucking at nothing while it looked from side to side and released short bursts of air and a few sparkling spit-bubbles.

Maybe you would half-smile and think, yeah, it's cute.

But after two seconds, you would have had enough and would be ready to go back to your desk, wondering why you didn't feel that irrepressible urge to gush.

Why you would keep hearing your own voice whispering, *Oh, hell no.*

You would eventually conclude that the kid thing just isn't for you.

If you're anything like me, you would feel a little excited by the discovery and, at the same time, maybe a little rebellious.

A *woman* who didn't want to have a *child*?

Most literature, movies, TV shows, and even news programs insist the exact opposite. Women want children so strongly we'll "try" for years, going as far as paying thousands of dollars to fertility clinics even if it means we could end up with septuplets. Or we'll adopt.

The extreme and mentally dysfunctional case of "I simply must have one" will kill a pregnant woman, slice open her abdomen, and steal the baby straight from her womb. You know you've seen it on *Lifetime*.

Even when the occasional storyline depicts a woman who claims to not want children, we soon find out she does, of course, secretly want them. Very much. But there's a reason she says she doesn't, and it's to protect herself psychologically. She either can't get pregnant and forces herself to believe she doesn't want to, anyway, or she is convinced she'll be a horrible parent (usually because she's had an abusive parent in her past, or she was orphaned and therefore had no "family" experience to pass onto her child). Ultimately, someone will convince her she'll make a fine parent, indeed, and by the end of the movie, she's getting an ultrasound.

But rarely will there be a woman who honestly, genuinely, and simply — without having to think about it for very long, if at all — has absolutely no desire to be a mother.

The absence of such characters in popular entertainment enforces the perception that women who don't want children aren't natural. That, as women, if we're not looking forward to being nurturers, there's something wrong with us, something different about us.

My friend D says, "It's also safe to assume that women who don't want kids are, in fact, in the minority, and that would be why they aren't represented as often. Just to be fair."

She's probably right, but unfortunately, being in the minority means not only being underrepresented, but also being susceptible to open criticism and judgment. You may have noticed people are much more comfortable with questioning women who don't want children than they are with questioning women who do want them (even if the women are clearly unfit).

In most movies starring women of childbearing age, if the women don't have children, it's usually because they a) are not yet married (most romantic comedies), b) are newly married and haven't had time to get pregnant (*Just Married*), c) are newly married and are actively trying to get pregnant (*She's Having a Baby*), d) had kids twenty years ago and the nest is empty (*The Big Chill*), or e) they're about to marry someone who has children of their own and will fit neatly into "motherhood" as a step-parent (*Step-Mom*).

The sooner women can confidently say "so what?" to not wanting kids, the sooner we'll stop struggling, stop trying to convince ourselves we *do* want them in a misguided effort to appease those who subscribe to the idea that childrearing is the one unquestionably acceptable route for women to take.

"Women, like men, are individuals," National Organization for Women co-founder Sonia Pressman-Fuentes said. "Some are suited to motherhood; others are not. Some want to work outside the home; others do not. Or women may want to do some of these things at certain times in their lives and not at others."

Okay, sure. We can be interested in careers and personal goals. But there should still be at least a *glimmer* of baby-interest hovering in the background, right?

No. *Not* right.

Stop thinking you're *supposed* to want them.

If there's very little you find enticing about spit-up and heavy diapers, accept it. Accept that you don't want to wake up for feedings or to a floor cluttered with toys. That you don't want to have to pack a diaper bag and ready a bottle and prepare a baby every time you leave the house. That you've seen those bathroom baby-changing stations and have walked by, almost every time, thankful to not have to deal with those contraptions and happy to be the one who gets to use the stall and leave, the only thing weighing down your arm a bag stuffed with new sweaters.

If one of the most restrictive futures you can imagine for yourself is one requiring babysitters, limited adult interaction, and conversations about diaper rashes and ointments and which baby said what word when and who's crawling, walking, or wearing colanders as hats, big deal. Accept that there's nothing wrong with not wanting to make dinner every night and breakfast every morning unless you're hungry, that not wanting your life as you know it to undergo an absolute and irreversible reconstruction is perfectly natural, and that being a mom simply isn't the life position you're looking to take on.

Accept that raising a child is just not your thing.

But do it without feeling like you're an unimaginably horrible person.

You don't have to want a baby.

THREE

TELLING PEOPLE

Every year as my dad's birthday approaches I'm a little more susceptible to the TV-commercial version of the parent-child relationship. The sweetness of a child sleeping on her father's chest. Sunlit mornings in the kitchen, mother and daughter sharing a bowl of sugar-free cereal.

Studio lighting and child actors have this way of filtering out reality, of dropping softened edges on parenthood to make it look suspiciously appealing.

But they don't blot out my own, unmediated visions of parenthood, which — before I decided I was absolutely not going to have children — came with panicky sensations akin to miniature minefields exploding under my ribs.

Then, one day, a baby appeared in one of my dreams.

It was a girl, and she wore a white, patterned jumper with booties attached to encase her feet. Her head rested on my shoulder, and I can still remember the weight of her plump, diapered behind on my arm. Her soft face was so close to mine I could smell it. Too, there was something about being unconditionally trusted, counted on, and required that was oddly appealing

There is no way for me to know the love a mother feels for her child, but that dream might have come close. It was one of the more intense and unique experiences I've had.

It was sweet.

It was nice.

Still, it was just a dream.

I've dreamed about many things, none of which, when I opened my eyes the next morning, seemed like quite as much fun in real life. Last night, for example, I had an exhilarating dream about being tossed into the ocean from the shiny, white wing of a passenger airplane.

Ten seconds of dream-inspired, warm baby feelings weren't quite convincing enough to cross the dream barrier into reality, and it was the inability of such a powerful and beautiful sensation to change my mind that clinched it.

I really just didn't want a kid. It was as simple as that.

I told Husband about the dream, shared the strange sensation of being what I imagined was a "mother," and then ended by stressing to him that I would really, honestly, very much hate to get pregnant.

We'd talked before about the slight possibility of a future with a child, and he'd been a little more open to the idea than I was. But any time we discussed it, if I said to him, "Okay. Well, do you want one right now?" he would say, "God, no!"

"Still," he would say. "I don't want to do anything permanent. What if? What if I change my mind? What if you do? You never know."

I would allow for that with, "Yeah, maybe."

(But, I did know.)

As time went on, and as we found ourselves having stronger and stronger aversions to all things parenthood — manifested as scowls at kids knocking down cereal boxes in the grocery store aisles, or as tight-lipped annoyance at child-heads popping up to make faces at us over the back of our chain-restaurant booth — it became pretty clear we were stepping ever further into the Non Parent (known today as DINK — Dual Income No Kids) demographic.

In fact, the older I got, the more I worried I might have twins if I got pregnant, or that I'd not only have a child, but also that my pregnancy would be high-risk and the baby would be born with an "abnormality," which meant it could require *extra* devotion, *extra* care, *extra* attention, and *extra* worry — none of which was something that interested me, since I wasn't even attracted to offering *regular* levels of devotion, care, attention, and worry. The only comfort I could take in the possibility of accidentally getting pregnant so late in life was that it had the potential to increase my risk of having a miscarriage.

(It should be noted that I am pro-choice. This is not synonymous with "pro-abortion" or "anti-life." Pro-choice means that if a woman, for reasons of her own, decides she will have an abortion, it is none of my business. It also means that I have the option to get an abortion, which, as I write this, is still a legal medical procedure. Although I am pro-choice, I do not relish the idea of having an abortion, myself. One of the reasons I don't want to have a baby, aside from the rearing, is that I don't want to be pregnant. I also don't want to give birth. It's not enough to not have children; the goal is to never get pregnant to begin with, and to never be in a position to consider abortion.)

A few weeks after the dream, Husband and I were sitting on the couch watching TV and groaning at a child actor intentionally acting like an annoying child.

I said, "Husband?"

"Hm?"

And then I said, "I really, really don't want kids. I'm over thirty. [*Which needs to be included, here, because for some reason no one really trusts decisions you make about having children until you're over thirty*]. I never wanted them before, and I'm not any closer to wanting them now."

And there.

It was out.

Decided-and-said to the person with whom offspring would or would not (in this case, not) be created.

It hadn't been telling him that had posed the problem; it had, I suppose, been voicing out loud, to someone — anyone — else, that I would *never* change my mind, and being prepared to accept any consequences.

It also meant not having to pretend, anymore, that I might consider, someday, popping out an offspring. The knee-jerk mutter that would come as a response to the question of children, *Yeahsure, maybesomeday*, could be permanently retired.

I imagine I felt the same way those who want children feel when they finally discover they're pregnant: successful. Something warm and electric spread through my chest and moved under my skin, made my hair follicles tingle. It was as if the heavy weight of the mere possibility of motherhood had mutated into its own heavy energy that, at that moment, simply lifted away from my body.

No

Children

!

Now that I'd told Husband, there was the question of whether we should tell others. After all, people who want children make any number of announcements:

"We want children."

"We can't wait to have children."

"We figure we'll wait a couple of years before we start having children."

"Oh, we want children right away."

"We've decided we're going to start trying."

"We're officially trying."

"John has a low sperm count, so..."

"We're going to specialists."

"We're pregnant!"

Whether you're single or in a relationship, someone will at one point invariably ask you — because your uterus hasn't yet been put to appropriate use — when you plan to have children.

Even if you're comfortable with not having them, you might still find yourself staring at the ceiling, pretending to think about it.

Well, I don't know, really … probably not before next week…

Maybe you'll shrug and say, "Well, I'm only thirty," which you'll immediately realize sounds ridiculous because one of your friends just a few years older than you has a twelve year-old and a ten year-old, and the other, who is your age, has two in daycare.

In fact, almost everyone your age has had kids for five to ten years, already.

So, you'll change your answer to, "I mean, what I mean is, I don't know," and you'll suddenly notice it's been some time since you've stirred the ice cubes in your glass. You'll stir them and, knowing they're still looking at you and waiting, you'll say, "In a couple of years, probably. You know. I don't know." You'll keep yourself from striking back with, *When are you going back to work?*

It's easier to pretend to want kids someday than it is to admit to not wanting them, because you're *expected* to want them some day. No one will question that decision. No one will say to someone who wants kids, "Aren't you afraid they won't come to visit you when you're old and alone in a nursing home?" or "Aren't you worried that five, ten years down the road you'll look back at your life and wonder whether you've lost yourself in your children?" No one will ask those questions because they're considered far less appropriate than those asked of people who don't want children.

Say you want children, and the conversation will move onto something else.

But say you don't want them, and an eyebrow will rise, or a drink will stop being drunk, or a mouth will open, or a forehead will fall.

"You *don't*?" they'll say, or, "Why?"

I used to be guilty of asking that, myself, but not because I thought women should have babies. It was because I wanted to know if their reasons were similar to mine. I stopped asking when, one time, the answer to "Why?" was "I can't."

It was a quick lesson in how personal a topic childbearing can be, and how frequently we take for granted that having children is simply something everyone can, and wants to, do.

Imagine a woman (not difficult, because we've all met this woman), a veritable stranger, who smiles and says enthusiastically to the clearly established couple, "So! When are we going to hear about a due date?" *Nudge, nudge, tickle, tickle the belly*, the Woman-As-Baby-Maker obviously public property.

Public Property says, "I'm barren."

Smiling, enthusiastic woman suddenly hushes and tightens her fingers around the stem of her white wine spritzer.

A "simple" question, in a moment, becomes impolite prying into what is possibly someone's personal trauma.

Unfortunately, that hasn't stopped people from asking, "Why no children?" and it likely never will. Consequently, whether or how to tell the people in your life you don't want children should be given some thought.

If you're going to be straightforward and say "No" or "Never" when people ask whether/when you're having children, expect to be asked to answer the follow-up, "Why not?" After answering it enough times, if you're spunky, you might make something up just to entertain yourself.

D, when she read the early draft of this very short ... book?, said that when she was pregnant she was infuriated that her womb seemed to be such a comfortable topic for others to discuss. She was surprised to learn a woman didn't necessarily have to be pregnant to have her uterus brought into a conversation.

"If I were childfree and people asked me such private questions," D said, "I'd probably tell them I was barren just to watch them squirm."

If, instead, you don't want to have fun and you're more comfortable being straightforward about your decision to not have children, be prepared to have the following conversation:

"Why don't you want kids?"

"I just don't."

"Why?"

You'll shrug.

"No, really. Did something happen?"

"Nothing happened." You might, for a moment, doubt yourself. Did something happen? "Like what?"

"I don't know. Were you abused?"

"No."

"You get along with your mom?"

"I get along with her just fine," you'll say.

"Was it your dad, then?"

"Was what my dad?"

"Was he distant? Never around? Working all the time?"

"No."

"Your mom. She's an alcoholic, right? Probably never showed you she loved you."

"She wasn't an alcoholic."

"Is she now?"

"No!"

"Really? Even with you not giving her grandchildren, and all?"

When I'm asked about children by acquaintances, my answer largely depends on mood. If I just want the conversation to stop short, "No immediate plans" is my stock answer. The assumption that I will someday be a mother is safe, then, and I've reassured someone with no stake in my life or the lives of my potential offspring that I, a walking uterus, will eventually undergo what looks like the excruciating hell of squeezing an entire person through my cervix in a room full of people staring at my vagina, and that afterward, I'll spend eighteen years to life caring for it.

Making an Announcement

Why make an announcement? Unless family members are bothering you for babies, there's no reason to share your personal decisions with them any more than there's a reason for them to pry into your intentions for your uterus.

FOUR

DEALING WITH THE OPPOSITION

One Thanksgiving evening, my dad and I sat on the patio of the house Husband and I mortgaged in New York. Husband was out flight instructing, and my dad and I were having a few drinks. As happens when conversations and drinks go long during festive holiday times, topics turned toward the more personal and we talked about kids and grandkids.

I was, after all, married.

Not only married, but married to the man I'd always wanted to be with. It was permanent, this time. It was real.

A long time ago, I'd told just about everyone — including myself — that if I were ever going to have a child, it would be with Husband.

That night outside with my dad, I told him that it was still true; if I were going to have a child, it would be with Husband.

But I still didn't think I'd have one.

He'd heard it all before, of course, when I was younger. When there was still time for me to change my mind. But when nothing changed from fifteen to eighteen to twenty-three to thirty years old, it finally registered with him that I might actually *not* have kids.

"Raising you girls," he said. "That's the best thing I ever did."

Then he called me selfish.

He didn't mean it in a bad way, even though it's almost impossible to not feel insulted after being called selfish.

He meant it as a statement of fact, and he was right.

I don't *want* my life to change. I don't *want* toys all over the place. I don't *want* to give up sleep. I don't *want* to worry. I don't *want* to feel the constant parental guilt that I'm somehow doing it wrong. I don't *want* other parents judging me for somehow doing it wrong. I don't *want* to put my goals on hold. I don't *want* to be pregnant. Most of all, I don't *want* to give birth. In that moment, life as a free-floating, unchained individual ends. Forever.

I don't *want* a newborn, a baby, a tot, a toddler, or a teen.

I, I, I...

Me, me, me…

But women who want children are selfish, too.

They want kids because they want them.

They want someone to love unconditionally.

They want someone to care for.

They want their genes to carry on.

They want to give someone a better life than they had.

They want to feel useful.

They want to create something that is the sum of the couple.

They want to solidify a relationship.

They want to make a husband stay.

They want someone to love *them* unconditionally.

They want a "Mini-Me."

They want to give their life a purpose.

There are just as many selfish reasons to have children as there are to not. What it boils down to is that parenthood is a life choice. A career-path. Or, for some, a calling.

Why would anyone do it if it didn't appeal to them? Propagation of the species, sure, but who's really thinking about that? Besides, it's not likely to be necessary for some time.

It boils down to desire. Personal choice.

Should a landscape artist at heart find a lifetime of work with an accounting firm?

"Stretch marks are the badge of a real woman."

In the movie "For Keeps," starring Molly Ringwald as a pregnant high school girl, she, her boyfriend, and their parents are arguing about the pregnancy when Ringwald's father hints that an abortion might be the best option. The boy's father, wide-eyed and red-faced, shouts over the voices of the arguing families, "Stretch marks are the badge of a *real* woman!"

Defining "womanhood" and "manhood" is a fun party game, but physical limitations aside, anyone can make and birth a baby. (If parents are reading this, I beg you not to take offense. I'm not saying "Parents are idiots." I wouldn't insult parents just to insult them — after all, I have two of them, myself.). A woman who fails to use birth control and lets the baby gestate and then gives birth to it is simply performing a task her body is physiologically equipped to perform.

"You have pets. You must want kids."

The following blog entry, written by radio and television producer and talk show host Linda Lowen, who specializes in women's issues, appeared online on October 19, 2007:

<u>Pets as a Substitute for Children?</u>

In the midst of the big fuss over Ellen Degeneres and her dog, I kept thinking that her situation is yet another example of a pet theory of mine: **Raising a dog or a cat is a trial run for raising children.**

...Is it selfish for a person or a couple not to have children? Many of us realize our capabilities and our limitations. Sometimes fur children are all that we can handle at a given point in our lives. But that doesn't diminish our commitment to them or our loving care. Yes, it does get crazy (not to mention expensive) when we carry them around in our handbags and dress them up in pricey outfits. But one person's love is another person's lunacy.

While the blog entry suggests that women who choose not to have children might simply be realizing their limited capabilities, or that animals are "all we can handle at a given point in our lives," both of which imply the decision to be childfree is indicative of some kind of personal shortcoming, it also likens pets to a gateway, of sorts, to parenthood.

A "trial run," she calls it.

Which may be true in some cases. Someone who can't handle the responsibility of a pet probably won't have much luck with children. On the other hand, I've known a few people who are completely inept in the pet department but who would undoubtedly make fabulous parents.

I have three cats, and I like them precisely because they're not children. They're cute, furry, small, don't speak human, and will never be teenagers. And my friends who have both children and pets will be the first to confirm that having a pet is nothing like having a child.

Instead of getting too deeply immersed into what is largely a bunch of supposition based on very little research and a lot of speculation, it seems simplest to say animals are not comparable to children any more than plants are comparable to pets. (Would you walk into someone's house, look at all of their plants, and say, "Hey, uh — why don't you just get a dog?")

FIVE

FINDING A MATE

You would think the absence of children in a relationship would *mean* the absence of children in a relationship, but apparently, they're part of it one way or another.

When you don't want kids, finding someone to be with long-term might not be as easy as it sounds. (Yes. I thought it would be easy. If you think it will be easy, don't.)

First, I should say Husband isn't someone I ended up with after launching an all-out quest for a husband who wouldn't try to get me to have babies. I've known him since we were in high school. I was the one to pursue him (bad girl—*The Rules* would not approve!) at seventeen. I saw him at school in the hallway, wooed him with my long, permed hair and pegged jeans, became the best of friends with him, and loved him evermore. It took more than a decade of bad timing and life separations to finally be together, and I consider myself extraordinarily lucky that the one person I most want to be with happens, by fortuitous coincidence, to not have that undeniable longing to be a parent.

I hate to think what it could mean for us if he did.

That said, I should also mention he's not the only person I've been married to, and that my feelings about parenthood contributed (in their own way) to the demise of my earlier relationships.

Popular culture would have us believe women are the baby-crazy sex, but a surprising number of men — as convincingly as sitcoms and movies about the Anti-Commitment Party-Men would argue otherwise — want families.

I thought a man who didn't want children should be an easy thing to find. In fact, I was certain there would be no need to actively look for one, that with so many of them out there, I'd just end up with one.

It didn't work out quite that way.

The more time I spent with male friends, the more hints they would reveal of daddy-in-the-making with off-hand remarks like, "When I have kids...," which takes for granted they'll have them. Someday.

A man who does not want children does not talk about his life and his future as if there will be children in it.

And a woman who doesn't want children has surprisingly few life-mate options, I discovered.

On the up side, we usually go through a few relationships before finding the right person, anyway, and not wanting children affords us the opportunity to have a clean breakup with little temptation to go back. Break-ups can get complicated when they're cluttered with differences in religious beliefs, career goals, and personal interests. Those are all things that can be *worked on*, and as a result, they contribute to the uncertainty people feel when they end a relationship. But the child argument is, if nothing else, one that cannot be solved unless someone gives in. When it comes time to end the relationship and move on, both parties in the break-up remain faultless, and because no one is being rejected for their personality, no one goes away feeling unloved.

But, oh, if you don't truly understand the depth and the strength of a person's desire to have children, it *is* easy to go away feeling angry.

-

I married for the first time at nineteen. Bill (whose real name is not Bill) and I were too young to get married, and we were also too young to know that before we married we were supposed to talk about things like religion, kids, finances, and anything else people planning to spend their lives together should know about one another.

The reason we didn't work out is simple: we weren't right for one another. In a number of ways. One of our differences was in the way we saw our future: he saw me having babies in it, and I didn't.

But that didn't come to the surface until later. Before we reached the period in our relationship when children would become an issue, we argued about other things. Most of our arguments were symptoms of our general unhappiness.

Now and then, I — young and passive-aggressive — thought about children, the fact that he wanted them, and the fact that my not wanting them would be a clean and clear way out. I wasn't ready to use it, yet, but I was well aware "I don't want kids" was, as a popular TV show host might call it, a deal-breaker.

When the final phase of our relationship came (the period during which at least one person in the relationship comes to accept the love, if it was love at all, is gone, and there's no salvaging it), I was scared to leave. What if we broke up, and then we realized we'd made the wrong decision? What if he ended up enjoying the separation and I didn't?

My mission was to stay until the relationship had been beaten so flat-dead that neither of us would experience a moment of regret at "goodbye."

So, I started fights.

Late one night, while Bill slept, I sat in the dark on the windowsill and smoked a cigarette. (This was back in the blissful time before I came to fear the dangers of smoking and could inhale deep and exhale slow and watch the smoke cloud form, then drift out the window, all without giving cancer or heart disease a thought. Good days.)

When the cigarette finished, I stubbed it out in the ashtray and climbed down from the cold sill. I walked across the bed on my knees and bounced until he looked like he was awake. I said, "Let's go on a trip somewhere."

Bill didn't open his eyes. "Hm?" he said.

"A trip," I said. "Let's just go somewhere. Anywhere."

"Like where?" He squinted, rubbed his forehead. "When?"

"I don't know where. And now. It's Saturday."

"You want to go somewhere now?"

"You don't?"

"Sylvia, come on. Don't do this."

"Don't do what?"

Of course, I knew perfectly well what I was doing. It may not have been as conscious a behavior as it seems to me now in retrospect, but I've no doubt that on some level two things were certain: he would say no, and I would have a reason to be disappointed in him.

Making someone else feel inadequate seemed to me an innocent enough effort, but because he didn't take the hint and leave me for it in a reasonable amount of time, enough time passed for me to see the effect it was having on him, and it dawned on me that I was actually being cruel.

The time had come to end things quickly, and permanently.

-

Bill had mentioned, in light conversation, that he wanted a house, a car, a wife, and kids. At nineteen, I was just learning what I wanted and didn't want, and I wasn't necessarily sure about most of my decisions. I wasn't positive at the time that I didn't want children, but I knew I didn't want them in that relationship.

So, I asked him to sit down. I told him I knew what he wanted.

"I just don't think we're going to work," I said, and he asked why. For reasons I'll never quite understand, he was unwilling to let go of us even when we were miserable. But it was time, and I would say the only thing I knew would work. "Even if we managed to fix everything else," I said, "I still wouldn't want kids."

Unexpectedly, this was ineffective.

He said we could talk about it. He said to give it some time, that maybe I would change my mind. We didn't have to have kids right then, after all. Who knew how I would feel at twenty-two or twenty-five?

After a few days, I brought it up again.

When that didn't work, I was annoyed. He didn't trust me. He didn't think I knew myself well enough to know I didn't want children.

The more people hear things, the more true those things become. So, whenever I was given the opportunity, I told him I didn't want children.

"What do you want for dinner tonight, Sylvia?"

"Chicken. You know I'm not changing my mind about kids, right?"

Bill was coming along in his own time, slowly (but surely) accepting he was as unhappy with me as I was with him. The Child Issue had started to move things along, and I was in a hurry for him to come around, to see things the way I did. I didn't want him to be sad about the breakup any more than I wanted to be sad, myself. It was important that he left knowing it was the right thing. Too, I was getting impatient. We'd already dragged it out far longer than we should have, and there was living to do.

I really wanted my own apartment.

Bill finally agreed: if I didn't want to have kids, he said, he didn't really see a future for us.

Now… Hold on a minute…

"So, wait," I said. "You say you love me, but then you tell me you only want to be with me if I'll make babies for you?"

This had not occurred to me before.

Why had this not occurred to me before?

My plan had seemed so simple until then. But now that it had actually worked, it felt a little too much like he was saying, *You're not enough by yourself.*

As much as I'd been counting on just that, it suddenly occurred to me that I meant less to him than a stranger, than some random woman he hadn't yet met who would give him a baby. I was *replaceable.* Our breakup based on differing views on procreation suddenly went from being no-fault to being very much his fault. It meant he had *lied* when he said he loved me. *He didn't know what love was* if he could toss me aside so easily for a woman he hadn't met and a maybe-someday baby who hadn't been born.

In the end, of course, we divorced — amicably — for all the right reasons, and there was no regret, on my part, about my decision to not have children. Having a baby with a person means accepting the person you're having a baby with will be in your life just as long as that child will, and not only did I not want children, but I also didn't want children with someone whose role in my life was temporary.

-

My relationship with Bill had taught me the value of discussing certain things with a mate before getting married. Like children. So before marrying next-husband Ted (whose real name is not Ted), I made sure to bring up the topic.

One night, while sitting at his table in his small attic apartment and holding the diamond ring he'd just given me, I said, "I probably might not want children, I don't think."

A box of mac and cheese waited to be cooked on his narrow, antique gas stove. Low music played from the living room, separated from the dining room by an imaginary line. Tall beer bottles lined a cabinet that acted as a wall between bedroom and living room, and records standing on end filled a cubbyhole shelf in the wall behind the couch.

It had been just a few minutes since he'd given me the ring. (The actual proposal had happened weeks prior in my own $125/month efficiency apartment.) I pinched the gold, beveled band between my fingers, made it flip back and forth under the light.

Sparkly.

I said, "I mean, I don't want you to go into this with the expectation that I'll have kids." To be perfectly clear, so he could not later claim to have been misled in any way, I added, "Even one kid."

"We don't have to have them," he said.

"Really?"

"If we have them, we have them. If we don't, we don't."

I believed him, and I was very excited.

But then, within two years, I discovered that at least one of us was, in fact, expected to have them. By that time, we'd talked about separation for unrelated reasons I later learned were actually related. (His desire to have children was a side-effect of his traditional upbringing, and the traditional upbringing explained his expectations of me and what he thought my role as his wife should be. It did not, however, explain what he must have been thinking when he told me he was okay with not having children. He later said, "I guess I thought you would change your mind.")

No one likes a breakup. It's painful. And Ted and I had started out as very good friends. That we were talking about separating made me sad, and even if it was the only thing left to do, I wasn't ready.

In a moment of desperation, I thought I might be able to not hate the idea of having a child.

For a brief second, I thought, "I guess I could want one…"

During that shortest of all seconds, I was on the couch in the living room of the house we rented. He sat at his desk in the dining room. We were divided by an open set of French doors.

"If you want a baby," I said, "now's the time."

His chair creaked when he leaned back to look at me. "What?"

"Now or never. If you want to have a kid, let's do it."

He sat there for a bit and then swiveled to face me. "Is this the right time?"

"They say there's never really a right time. You just do it."

"I don't know, Sylvia," he said.

He went on to say more things, and somewhere in the middle of his protests, I stopped listening because I was preoccupied with *holyshitwhatthewhatdidIjustsay?* relief that he'd hesitated, that I wasn't at that moment being impregnated.

Humoring wild impulses that have life-changing consequences cannot be a good idea.

(The impulse returned only once, and that was the year Husband was doing the war thing. Afraid he might die, I thought having his child might be the only way to keep a part of him with me if he didn't come back.)

As time passed after my spontaneous offer of motherhood, and as I became even more certain I didn't want to have kids, we decided to separate. It was after the separation that he admitted he really had always hoped I would change my mind about children.

I felt lied to.

Betrayed.

And, once again, as if I'd been reduced to a baby-making machine.

Luckily, as mentioned earlier, we'd already reached a point in our relationship when we were talking about separation for a variety of relationship-killing reasons. Our child disagreement simply made it easier for both of us to call it over. There was no amount of therapy, talking, wanting, rethinking, or wishing that could make us stay even a week longer. There was no point.

What I understand now, and what my need to feel *done wrong* and *wounded* had me refusing to understand then, is that someone's desire to have a baby is just as strong as someone's desire not to. If something extraordinary isn't keeping two people together, it's no easier for a person who wants children to stay child-free with someone than it is for someone who has never wanted children to imagine having one they don't want — even if what's between the two is something close to real love.

Of course, that's just been my experience.

"Finding a mate" is this chapter's title. I can't tell you how to find a mate, but I can tell you to try to avoid the potential mates who want children. You might be able to get them to agree to live child-free, but you'd be running the risk of being the cause of a lot of resentment. There's also the risk of having to watch him look wistfully at passing mothers with their children.

"Why can't *you* do that?" you'd hear him thinking.

"Look how beautiful mothers are," you'd read into the look he gave the rosy-faced woman with a small hand yanking hers.

"Look how perfect pregnant women are," you'd label the sigh, attributing it to adoration and wonderment as you pass a waif with a basketball belly pushing taut a pair of denim overalls.

At the work party, when his friend Bob would talk about his wife's pregnant glow, you'd hear him thinking, "*My* wife doesn't glow."

This is not to say that's what he would, in fact, be thinking, but it would be hard not to wonder.

There's also the risk of the relationship falling apart ten years down the road when he frees himself to have kids while he still can.

The best you can do is be straightforward and clear. Say you don't want kids. Tell the men in your life you don't see yourself changing your mind.

When they say, "But it's possible you will," only you'll know what to say. (You must have something in mind for that one.)

And, when you find yourself married to someone who wants kids and you don't — which probably happens often, as women are expected to change their minds — and you reach that impasse that results in an end, don't take it personally.

Try not to, anyway. It's not about you. If you got pregnant and had the baby and became a mom, remember, that problem would be solved and the relationship probably wouldn't end. (At least, not because of your reluctance to have children.) Then again, you'd have that baby and everything that comes along with it...

SIX

MAKING IT HAPPEN

It should be simple to *not* have children. In fact, much of the literature on getting pregnant makes conception seem dauntingly difficult.

First, the egg has to be produced. Then it has to be released and travel through the fallopian tube. The sperm has a key window of opportunity — just a few days in any given month — to reach and fertilize the egg. But, for the sperm to do that, it has to not only arrive in the fallopian tube while the egg is there, but it has to *get* there.

For the sperm to get there, the man has to ejaculate enough semen to deliver the sperm, and the sperm itself has to be the right shape and size and even move the right way. Of 300 million sperm on their way to the egg, about 200 reach it. Not 200 million — two hundred.

Books upon books, articles upon articles, instruct women how to get pregnant.

But, what if you don't want to get pregnant and you're not in a committed relationship with a man willing to get a vasectomy (a far less invasive, and more effective, procedure than anything that is surgically done to a woman)?

Many doctors will refuse to perform tubal ligations on women under 30. "Though no actual laws have ever been put into place, most OBGYNs refuse to provide women under thirty with permanent forms of contraception," writes Bonnie Zylbergold in her 2007 article "Are You Kidding?"

The article goes on:

With thirty plus years of medical practice, Dr. Wiener finds no good reason for putting otherwise healthy patients in surgery: for one, there are anesthetic risks involved. Plus, tubal ligations are considered elective surgeries (assuming the patient can use other, less invasive forms of birth control). More pressing, still, is the fear that a patient may one day change her mind.

In other words, they want to protect women from themselves.

If you decide you want your tubes tied, and if you *still* want to have them tied after educating yourself on the associated risks, it might involve a lengthy, frustrating search, but you'll probably eventually find a doctor who trusts you to make your own decisions about your life. One who recognizes that by not deciding for you that you might want children some day, you are being allowed to take the responsible avenue: protecting yourself from an unwanted pregnancy rather than risking getting pregnant, and then perhaps being put in a position to decide whether to get an abortion or put the baby up for adoption. Or, obviously, keep it.

People who don't want children generally don't even want to be pregnant, so there's very little about an accidental, unwanted pregnancy that isn't accompanied by unpleasantness. That there are people out there waiting desperately to adopt the baby is a minuscule comfort when compared to how great it would have been to not get pregnant in the first place.

I read somewhere, once, something by a woman who said she refuses to have sex until she's had a tubal ligation.

Smart woman.

But, most of us don't have that self-restraint. Ideally, I suppose we would, and maybe it's something of a copout to say that, to some degree, we're just animals. Just creatures. We have sex drives and very little self-control, most of the time, and if most doctors won't perform a tubal ligation until the patient is 30 or older ... well, you do the math.

It's hardly realistic to expect all women who don't want children to remain abstinent either until they're

30, or until they can not only afford a tubal ligation but find a doctor willing to do it.

Which makes staying child-free difficult and stress-filled. Until someone has had an operation — either you, or the man you're having sex with — there's always that nail-biting wait as it gets closer and closer to the time your period is due.

Here's why there's nail-biting even if you're pretty sure you're being careful (information comes directly from statistics listed on Planned Parenthood's website, www.plannedparenthood.org):

Condom use: Each year, 2 out of 100 women whose partners use condoms will become pregnant if they **always** use condoms correctly. Each year, 15 out of 100 women whose partners use condoms will become pregnant if they **don't always** use condoms correctly.

Implanon: Less than 1 out of 100 women a year will become pregnant using Implanon.

IUD: Less than 1 out of 100 women will get pregnant each year if they use the ParaGard or the Mirena IUD.

The pill: Less than 1 out of 100 women will get pregnant each year if they **always** take the pill each day as directed. About 8 out of 100 women will get pregnant each year if they **don't always** take the pill each day as directed.

The shot: Less than 1 out of 100 women will get pregnant each year if they always use the birth control shot as directed. About 3 out of 100 women will get pregnant each year if they don't always use the birth control shot as directed.

The percentages seem small, sure. No reason to worry.

Until, I imagine, you're the one making up that small percentage.

People get pregnant all the time. Why shouldn't it be you?

As unrealistic as it might be to abstain from sex to avoid pregnancy, unless you're permanently fixed, it really is the only sure-fire method.

The point is, whether you end up pregnant is largely up to you. (I say "largely" because you can hardly be blamed for a pregnancy that occurs after you, or your partner, has had an operation to prevent such a thing.)

In short, here are your choices:

Don't have sex.

Be diligent about taking birth control.

Use a secondary measure.

Use a third measure.

Get an operation.

If he never wants children, discuss his thoughts on having a vasectomy (the procedure is less involved than a tubal ligation, and men generally experience far fewer risks and side-effects).

Or, do none of the above and hope for the best, and then kick yourself when you discover you're with child

-

Another key to making a child-free life happen is not allowing yourself to be bullied by people who think you should have kids.

"Bullied" might be too strong a word, but small suggestions here and there, little nudges over the years, and the barrage of not-too-subtle suggestions from the media (whether produced for entertainment value or in the form of endless literature instructing women how to have children while young, while old, while already caring for multiple children, while divorcing, while married, while gay, or while a woman who wants to raise a baby without a male partner) that women-have-babies-that's-just-what-women-do, can feel like bullying.

We're taught when we're young not to succumb to peer-pressure, and there's no reason that should change as we get older. Just because all of your friends and a huge percentage of strangers are doing it doesn't mean you have to. In fact, doing something because other people do it just means you've become a victim of a popular fallacy, the bandwagon appeal.

The bandwagon appeal is a popular tactic used by politicians, advertisers, and pretty much anyone else who wants to either rationalize or encourage behavior.

Parent to child: "What is this? Pot? Pot! Marijuana! Right there in your drawer! Why would you have drugs in your drawer?"

Child: "Aw, c'mon, Dad. Everyone does it."

When I was twelve, the boy I had a crush on decided to bring a box of beer to school. He'd packed beer bottles wrapped in T-shirts in a box and brought them on the bus we rode together.

I asked him for one. Not to impress him, but to do something I wasn't supposed to be doing.

He took out a bottle and gave it to me, and I remember drinking about a third of it. (I never did develop a taste for beer, as many years as I tried.)

During second period, I was called to the principal's office. The boy had been caught with the box of beer, and he'd caved, had given up my name to reduce the trouble he was in.

I was suspended for the rest of the day, and I had to call my dad and not only tell him why I was suspended, but ask him for a ride to the train station so I could get home.

On the way there, my dad said, "Why'd you drink the beer?"

I told him the truth. "I just wanted to."

He didn't believe me, so he asked me again. *Why did you drink the beer? You couldn't have done it for no reason. No one drinks beer before seven in the morning without a reason. Or without being an alcoholic, and I know you're not an alcoholic.*

It became clear that he needed me to have a reason. He—even after all of his instructions about being independent and not letting the behavior of others dictate what we do—actually *wanted* me to have been pressured into it. That seemed strange to me at the time, because it struck me as the favoring of weakness over strength, but considering the behavior he wanted an explanation for, I figured it made a certain kind of sense.

The reason he extended to me sounded good, so I used it.

"I wanted to be cool," I told him.

Immediately, he relaxed. His mood lightened, he talked more, and he even gave me money for the train when he dropped me off. "Do something useful with your day," he said when I opened the door to get out, "and be good."

If the bandwagon appeal weren't so cunningly effective, trends wouldn't exist.

But it's no reason to have a baby.

What happens after the cave-in? After you get 'er done, get pregnant, and do what you suppose you're supposed to be doing?

Well, you take that baby home and raise it for eighteen years or more, that's what. Those people you perceive as pressuring you certainly won't do it for you. TV won't do it, actors won't do it, and your friends won't do it.

In fact, most of them won't even know you were ever pregnant. As strong as the subtle nudges from society can feel at times, they don't know you. Not your name, not your marital status, not your goals, not your plans. They truly have no influence over you whatsoever, so allowing invisible pressures to push you into thinking you're supposed to be a parent even if you don't want to be will probably do little but help you think, "At least I won't feel like I'm being looked at funny, anymore."

But you'll still have that baby to raise for the next eighteen years. Or more.

SEVEN

SOCIAL AWKWARDNESS
(OR, BEING THE ONE CHILD-FREE ADULT IN THE ROOM)

One fall day, Husband and I had dinner on a balcony restaurant on a shop-lined street. Space heaters set up outside were almost warm enough. We'd had a good day walking around and studying sculpted cows bolted to the sidewalk, each painted with a different motif. One was white with blue flowers, another had painted-on overalls and boots, even an iPod in a worn shirt pocket.

We waited for our food, watching the sun drop, and a nicely-dressed man, close to our age and carrying an equally nicely-dressed toddler, came through the door and brought his boy to the railing so, together, they could look down at the street.

The kid wore a big, wool sweater and khaki pants and boots. His style matched his father's fitted leather jacket and slacks, shoes with little wear, and heavy knit sweater.

We noticed their clothes, the way the two matched, and commented (aside) on the cuteness of the boy. After they left and were replaced by another parent close to our age coming up to the balcony with a kid to look out at the sunset and down at the street, we whispered, "Everyone has kids!"

Maybe not everyone, but certainly more people in their thirties have kids than don't. My two best female friends have children, two each. The women I know who don't have kids are still in their early twenties and "don't want them yet, but some day—don't you?"

Husband's male friends all have two or more children.

In Hollywood, babies are being born to women twenty, thirty, forty years old. Every month, some new actress is pregnant. Married actresses, single actresses, actresses recently caught driving the wrong way on the interstate after taking too many drugs with their alcohol, even the sixteen year-old actress-sister of a twenty-something singer who almost lost her own kids after proving to be not such a hot parent.

They're everywhere, babies.

Going to most social functions after a certain age (say, 25) means being surrounded by people who are "grown-ups" or "adults" who've hired babysitters for the night and can't stay long. When they get home, they'll check on the kids. They're adults the same way my

father is still an adult to me, and the same way my
teachers and my friends' parents were "grown-ups"
when I was a kid. They're the *others.* The establishment.
Which is strange, because looking at them when they're
not with their children is like looking at playmates.
They're the same age, which means they look "young,"
and not "old" the way, as a child, frumpy old parents
looked to us. But when it's revealed the people who look
like us have children, there's a moment of "Oh..." before
their faces almost immediately and magically transform
into the Father or Mother look so often picked out by
commercial producers looking for men and women to
play the parent role in air sanitizer or vacuum cleaner
ads.

At a party, surrounded by people who are parents, I
wonder, sometimes, if they might be watching me the
way adults watch children, waiting for me to stick my
finger in someone's dip or for my shoelace to come
untied. Parents have something different about them.
Something ... paternal. A certain inflection in their voice
that, were you to hear it, would automatically leave you
standing at attention and no longer doing whatever it
was you were doing.

"Jennifer."

"Yes!" You'll drop the water cracker on the platter
and wonder how many you'd already eaten. *Had you
been hogging the crackers?* Had *you?*

-

When we lived in New York, while Husband was in the military, I made contact online with a woman who had just moved to the area with her military husband. We were both friendly enough with one another at first, asked "Where'd you come from?" and "What brought you here?" questions in our emails. Then the woman told me she had three children and asked, "Do you have kids?"

I wrote back that, no, I didn't.

I didn't hear from her again.

Not being a mother often means not only being the odd woman out, but it also strips you of a ready conversation piece when thrust into the company of strangers.

Mothers, it seems, can bond almost immediately simply by talking about their children. Even if there's no plan to become friends, when happenstance sticks them in a room together, even if one has pink, spiked hair and a nose-ring, even if the other is tucked safely in a chaste pink sweater set, even if they have nothing to say to one another about anything else while munching water crackers at the snack table, there's always Johnny's tendency to tie his shoelaces to chair legs or Jenny's cute way of eating butter sticks with a spoon.

The women's glaringly obvious differences are irrelevant; their children are a common link helping them avoid the awkwardness of being silent.

Without kids, though, as the one who just wants to grab a snack but feels obligated to be social, that conversation can be like watching a slow game of golf on TV. Every now and then, punk-mother might chip an eagle with a cute story and you'll find yourself laughing or saying, "Aw," but when the topic shifts to good teachers versus bad teachers and good districts versus bad districts and which diapers absorb more and smell less, it can be like watching golfers walk 300 yards on a fairway. Oh-my-yawn.

Talk of such things is undoubtedly fascinating if you're a parent. I know I'd have opinions on everything from booties to teething toys if I were a parent.

But as a non-parent?

A non-parent is eternally the child. The only experience with parenthood non-parents have is that of having parents; therefore, the stories we can tell are those empathizing with the children. The best we can do if we want to contribute is say, "Oh, I remember when I did things like that. My parents wanted to kill me." And then we'll nod and blow air through a straw into a soda glass.

A few years ago, I visited D, who's been in my life since we were nine years old. When I visited, her daughter was seven, the boy, ten.

During my visit, I went along with D to take her kids to Sunday school. The drive was accompanied by constant chatter from backseat to front, little voices saying very important things into the air, some of which got a response from mom, some of which didn't.

After dropping them off, we had about an hour before it would be time to go back and pick them up. I thought it would be a chance for D to have a rest, but in that hour, D dropped off movies, did laundry, and picked up the house. After getting the kids, it was time to take them to their martial arts class. The boy was an active participant, but it was the little girl's first time and she was shy and didn't want to participate.

D, to encourage her daughter, got out there and did the exercises. She crawled around the room on her hands and knees, performed the defensive moves demonstrated by the instructor, and jumped over a stack of plastic bricks, back and forth, back and forth. All the while watching her daughter, coaxing her to join.

Her daughter didn't join.

The class ended, D thanked the instructor for being so patient, and we went back to her house, where she urged her kids to play in their bedroom. On her short break, she made us some coffee and we stood drinking it in her kitchen.

Rather, she stood still for about two minutes before pulling food from the refrigerator and plates from the cabinets and making lunches. She had three sips of coffee the whole time, and popped the mug in the microwave every now and then because she was too occupied to enjoy it while it was hot.

I used to wonder what a stay at home mom did all day. I thought, "I know it's busy, but it can't be busy all the time. Surely they have at least three hours a day (right there—if you're a stay at home parent, you're laughing hysterically at 'three hours') to pop in a DVD, or play around on the computer. *Something*."

That day with D, I learned. Her life exhausted me. I was constantly amazed by her sweet demeanor toward her very cute son and daughter who, cute as they were, absorbed what seemed like all of her time. I groan if someone calls me when I'm not in the mood to talk on the phone, so how did this woman tend to other people all day long?

She's cut out for it. That's what it is. And she loves it. She truly loves being a mother to her son and daughter, and that's why she's so good at what she does, why it doesn't drive her crazy.

We continued to work on the coffee while she busied herself with heating and preparing food until it was time to call the kids down for lunch. She had them sit at a child-sized table in the middle of the kitchen and set their plates in front of them.

Then she handed me a plate she'd made for me.

She squirted ketchup on her own plate, her son's plate, her daughter's plate.

And then she squirted ketchup on my plate.

I looked at it.

"Oh my god," she said, and laughed. "I don't know why I did that. I know you can do your own ketchup." She was still laughing when she said, "Habit."

If ever I feel too much like a grown-up, I'm driving to D's house so she can make me lunch and squirt ketchup on my plate.

-

Someone I was involved in a discussion with recently said he believed childless people to be "relatively carefree."

In response, another man, this one in a DINK relationship, said, "Kid-free does not, by any means, mean 'carefree'."

I was tempted to agree. "It certainly does not mean carefree," I almost replied with what I thought was probably justifiable indignation. "We people with no kids to take to the hospital, or to buy clothes and groceries for, have plenty of cares and our share of very serious concerns. You want a list of mine? I'll make you a list."

Too often, and too easily, being child-free—because of the unfounded, society-induced guilt associated with it—means there is an instinct to *defend! defend! defend!* against what seem like accusations.

How responsible could you be if you're not caring for children? If you don't have children, what do you do all day? What, you just get up, go to work, and go home? And then what? Watch TV?

A few years ago, a man suggested that because I didn't have a full-time job or children to take care of, I should have had plenty of time to make complicated meals from scratch to save in the freezer for future meals instead of buying the mass-produced, frozen dinners I was buying.

It was hard not to spit out a list of any one of my days' activities that left me with very little time to do anything else. Even now, as I write this, I'm tempted to write exactly what it was I was doing at the time that kept me so busy that taking just five minutes to microwave a version of ravioli felt like a huge cut into a tight schedule. Lunch was a necessity, not a welcome break, and it was often skipped because it knotted my rhythm.

But what I was doing when I wasn't raising children or ripping carrots out of the ripe earth or butchering my own cow for stew doesn't matter.

The only thing that kept me from giving him that list was that it would have been the same as saying there was something to defend.

You've heard that the more money people have, the more they spend. It's probably the same with time. The more time we have, the more ways we find to fill it with things.

Instead of driving kids to and from soccer practice, maybe time is spent getting a coffee in a café downtown. Or doing leftover work. Or taking a yoga class. Or playing hockey. Or writing essays, learning to play drums, donating time to charities, refinishing furniture, weaving baskets, taking flight lessons, writing bad poetry … etc.

Learning to play drums … taking yoga … writing bad poetry…

Wait a minute.

Aren't child-free adults, in fact, at least a little more carefree than parents?

Well, sure. But isn't that, at least in large part, the point?

EIGHT

THEY'RE NOT JUDGING JUST YOU

Joan Chrisler said there are several negative stereotypes attached to women who don't want children: they're cold; they hate children; and/or they're selfish.

"The reaction I hate the most is when people ask me, 'How does your husband feel about you not having children?'" says Phoena G., a 35-year-old woman who runs a website called "Happily Childfree." Phoena says she is insulted by the implication that she requires her husband's approval to remain childfree, or that she's somehow cheating her husband out of his "rightful children."

Regardless of what might be a negative perception of childfree women, N.O.W. co-founder Sonya Pressman-Fuentes said the choice to have or not have children is a boon to women and their families.

"Women today have the opportunity to reach their maximum potential" as career women, wives, or mothers, she said.

Chrisler said even romantic relationships have been proven to benefit from being childfree. Not only is there less stress caused by sleeplessness and errand-running, but couples without children have more money to spend on fun activities because they're not saving for college tuition and weddings for their children.

"It's absolutely true," says my friend T, a 35-year-old Minnesota mother to a son, a daughter, and a step-daughter. "Being in a second marriage and choosing not to have children with my husband now, we do have a lot more money for fun activities."

But even mothers aren't free from judgment by other mothers. T, while expressing how much she enjoys the time she gets to spend with her husband during the summers when her children leave to visit their father, reiterates (again and again) that she loves her children and wouldn't trade them for anything. As if she's been conditioned to do it.

"I got a dirty look from someone the other day at work when I said I love my summers," she says. "She was like, 'Don't you miss your kids?' Yes, I miss my kids desperately, but when they go to their father's I don't have to do their laundry, or do their dishes, or drive them places. I take advantage of things I don't get to do normally, like things with my husband. We can hang out on the couch."

And sleep in.

While I'll not deny we child-free types do face some judgment and criticism, and although, as women, we're marginalized when it comes to choosing the best juices ("As a mom, I want to know my juice is all natural," one commercial advertised – do we non-moms not want natural juice, too?) and receiving special labels ("Coma Mom Defies the Odds,"a recent morning show episode headlined—is she somehow special because she's a mom, and not just a woman, who defied the odds?), I think we have it easier than moms do, and not just because we don't task ourselves with raising children.

Don't misunderstand—women who are uncertain about whether they want to have children, or who have just realized they'll never want them, have a tough time, for a while. Deciding not to have children means being something of a social outcast, experiencing some difficulty finding a life partner, and periodically wondering whether being child-free was the right choice. The child-free also have to deal with guilt-trips from parents and in-laws who want grandchildren, the constant barrage of "Aren't you afraid you'll regret it?" and "What happens when you're old and alone?" questions, and feeling like society believes we're "unnatural," in general (because everyone knows it's "natural" to want, and have, children).

Even so. I'd much rather suffer whatever judgment I might receive as a child-free woman than what I suspect I'd have to deal with if I were a mother.

For instance, if you type "should mothers" into the Google search bar, the options it will bring up for you automatically include "stay at home," "work," "sleep with their children," and "work outside the home."

And if you type "mother's shouldn't" into the search bar, the auto-suggestions are "work," "Facebook," and "have Facebook." (Really? People are discussing whether mothers should be on Facebook?)

Other questions people ask about mothers (and many of them make the morning show segments) include:

- Is it okay for mothers to have a glass of wine during playdates with other mothers?

- Should mothers breastfeed?

- How long should mothers breastfeed?

- Should mothers breastfeed in public?

- Should mothers give their children milk?

- Should older mothers be allowed to have more children?

- Should mothers have more than one child?

And that's just conversation taking place in the media. Mothers (*after* being touched on their pregnant bellies by strangers) also have to deal with other mothers. Other mothers, who are certain they're raising their own children the right way, are often the first to criticize the way other mothers raise their children:

"Really? You let them eat that?"

"Really? You let them watch that?"

"Really? You let them listen to that?"

"Oh, you don't make him do his homework as soon as he comes home?"

"You let her boyfriend go into her bedroom?"

"You don't go to every single soccer practice?"

"You let him have coffee? Really? At fifteen?"

"You bought condoms for her? Really? At fifteen?"

"You let her wear that?"

"You don't let her wear that?"

"Wait – you went OUT?"

We all have our issues where children (or a lack thereof) are concerned, but I'm willing to bet my early years of non-mom guilt, two divorces, and pregnancy fears as a child-free woman were far more tolerable than it would have been to hear one single unsolicited word about how I was raising my child. (And I'm pretty certain mothers have to deal with this for the full eighteen years. There are "right" ways to care for infants, toddlers, pre-teens, teens...)

A note: This should not be confused with something that turns mothers into heroes. It isn't, and they aren't. ("Hero" is a word that should be reserved only for those who risk their lives for others even as they fear for themselves.) Nor should it be mistaken for something that minimizes the experiences of the child-free. It is simply an attempt at an honest assessment of the judgment women receive (and cast) under the category "childbearing." (There are many other categories under which women are judged, but we see those every day in magazine and television ads.)

NINE

DON'T FEAR THE QUESTION

That cute kid with his father overlooking the shopping district from the balcony restaurant...

He wasn't the only one to make it possible to imagine having one of my own little people walking next to me on the sidewalk, small hand in my fingers.

There was also this amazing red-headed girl.

Husband and I saw her on the shuttle from the airport to the parking lot after a vacation one summer. It was just her mother, her father, and her. She, this tiny person, sat on the bench between her mom and dad, who allowed her to sit independently. Their hands were just close enough to grab her if she leaned precariously. This girl, who wasn't old enough to walk but who was old enough to sit on her own, watched and watched. Watched everything.

Babies usually tend to look around like everything is new, like every shiny, colorful object requires inspection. This little girl seemed to have seen it all before.

She was incredible.

She was quiet, adorable, and — Husband and I were convinced — a genius.

"If we ever had one," I said to Husband, "I'd want her to be like that."

"I know!" he said.

We play the 'if' game a lot.

"If we had kids, they'd get a used beater when they turned sixteen, not some new car."

"If we had a daughter, she would *not* wear shirts like that."

"If we had a son, he would not wear pants with the waist down past his butt."

"Our kid wouldn't get a laptop for Christmas."

"Our kid would have to work to pay her own cell phone bill."

"If our kid threw a tantrum in a grocery store, we'd leave him there."

Not having children affords us the freedom to make our hypothetical child anything we want. When she's bad, she's disciplined. When she won't be disciplined, she's sent to boot camp where she's forced to walk in the rain or wear unstylish jeans and sneakers. A week later, our daughter may be a son, and not only is he washing cars for free all day Saturday after he's caught speeding down a residential street, but later that night, he's doing all the dishes along with anything else parents make kids do to help them "learn responsibility"/give the parents a rest.

Of course, not having real children also means we don't need that rest and don't have to deal with the headache of actual discipline.

When we play the kid game, I still — every now and then — get a little uncomfortable, because I am more anti-parenthood than Husband is. If I wanted to, say, adopt a child some day, he would be willing to consider it.

On the other hand, if he told me he would like to have a child some day, I can't say I would be as open to the idea.

When we play the hypothetical child game, I sometimes wonder if there's a part of him that wants a child. I wonder if that little part will creep to the surface years and years from now and retroactively resent me for not having one.

He says if he wanted children, he would tell me.

I trust him to tell me the truth, so I believe him.

And I hope he doesn't change his mind.

Because he had once considered having children in his past, for me to accept that I don't want children means I also have to accept there is the slightest possibility my relationship with him could see a serious conflict in the future, should he — for whatever reason — decide not having children was the wrong thing to do.

I knew a woman, once, who didn't want children, but who had them anyway because she loved her husband.

I am not that woman. As much as I love Husband, I would never have children just to make him happy.

Obviously, I can't see the future and therefore can't say with 100 percent certainty that I'll never change my mind (things happen; family members die and leave babies behind, a child could somehow be presented to me as one in dire need), but I can say it with as much confidence as I can say, "I will never intentionally pick up a gun and kill a non-rabid kitten."

At some point, we just know ourselves, don't we?

Often, however, people who don't want children are still posed with the question of possible regret.

"What about when you're seventy and have no one left around you? Wouldn't you want family to visit you? Children to care for you?"

"Aren't you afraid you'll regret not having children?"

The nice thing about regret and child-freeness is that if at some point I regret not having a child, I can probably find a way to have one. Options range from adoption to foster care to hiring a surrogate mother.

On the other hand, let's say I had a child simply to avoid the possibility of future regret. Not only does that not strike me as a good foundation for parenthood, but what would my options be if I ended up regretting having the child I didn't really want and only had so I could try to avoid regret?

I have a feeling it's easier to install a new child into a life than it is to remove one from it.

And if my only regret about not having children when I'm old is that I should have had one so I'd have a sometimes-visitor to keep me company during game shows, that would simply confirm I was right not to have one.

And then there's this question: "But, what'll happen to the human race if everyone stops having children?"

That is the question of an alarmist. It's highly improbable that every woman on the planet will simultaneously decide they don't want children.

-

Major life decisions come with doubt — it's part of the deal. People who have been married for years still sometimes wonder if they made the right choice, or what their lives might have been had they run from the altar at the last minute and lived a single life.

"I could be in Zimbabwe or Tibet right now," they're thinking while watching a rerun of "Everybody Loves Raymond."

Those who didn't marry the one they really wanted to ten years ago probably still wonder, now and then, "What if I had?" and study the one they did marry, then turn off "Everybody Loves Raymond" because, hey, they're living it — why watch it on TV?

A homeowner grumbles about the house she bought when the rain gutter fills and drops. Someone fifteen years into her career wonders if maybe she should have done what she always wanted to do and opened that store selling natural fiber products. Someone else who owns such a store pauses for a moment and regrets owning her own business, longs for just one weekend of not worrying the business will fail, and then goes back to counting inventory.

The next morning, though, the one who didn't run from the altar throws a leg over her husband and hugs him for being nothing like the character of Ray Romano. The other married woman still wonders what it would have been like to marry the guy she didn't (sometimes, the grass really *is* greener on just one side). The woman who grumbled at her rain gutter sits on her patio and watches a blue jay perch on the birch tree she planted in the corner of her yard. The woman fifteen years into her career thrives on the work she's doing and takes pride in the success she's had, and the store owner unlocks the door to her shop and breathes in the smell of cotton, hemp, and her creation.

Likewise, a parent watching her child throw a fit over a timeout laments the day of that child's conception, and a non-parent envies a smile shared between a father and son.

The next day, the parent holds the child in front of a winter window and smells freshly shampooed hair.

The non-parent walks around naked with a cup of coffee before getting dressed to do anything she wants for the day.

When smiling at the cuteness of a child elicits the reaction, "Are you *sure* you don't want kids?" I am tempted to save for the day she rolls her eyes or grits her teeth at being overly busy or stressed, "Are you sure you should have had yours?"

Whether you're sure you don't want children is a question that is, or should be, only yours to ask of yourself.

Without the question, how can there be an answer?

It seems it can only be healthy to check in every now and then, even if the answer is a given. Is there a time when self-exploration should end?

Even if you've decided and accepted that you don't want children, you might still find you ask yourself, "Am I sure I don't want kids?" Particularly when you see one that strikes you as what is probably an ideal child who you imagine is never a bother and, somehow, feeds and clothes herself or otherwise just sits around being cute.

The question doesn't have to be threatening. When I ask myself "Are you sure?" it just means I'm exploring and considering one of the many avenues that won't be taken, because I've chosen another. We can't do everything. We have to pick and choose. We do our best.

Probably the most powerful, and unexpected, experience I've had in terms of questioning the decision came after the choice had been irrevocably (for the most part) made, surgically speaking. I was very excited when Husband told me he would get a vasectomy, so you can probably imagine my surprise when shortly after he had the operation and our child-free life together was guaranteed, I was so sad I almost couldn't stand it.

It had to be the fact that I was no longer worried about the possibility of pregnancy that "what-if" scenarios, which were no longer a direct threat to me, had an entirely new face.

Suddenly, I was thinking of all the times I'd seen him interact with children (the ones he liked, anyway); he was so natural, so fun. He's the kind of person who says off-the-wall things to kids that I would never think to say in a million years because I just don't "get" kids, that way. I remembered how much the children of a friend of ours latched onto him, the little girl in particular. (I can't say that I blame her.) Everywhere he went, she went.

And here he was, now, never to have children of his own. I couldn't help but think I had done some unborn child the greatest disservice imaginable by depriving them of this beautiful, generous, kind, funny, understanding man as a father, and it was killing me.

That I told him all of this while he was still sensitive from being tugged and cauterized might not have been the best decision, timing-wise. He didn't say much. I still don't know what he was thinking that day. It probably sounded a little bit like, "Are you ____ing crazy? I just had this done and now you don't want it?" That's what I would have been thinking, were I him, so I assured him (while crying all over him) that I didn't regret the decision. I still didn't want children, and I never would. "You'd just make such a good dad," I bawled.

I suppose it hit me in a way it hadn't before that it wasn't only my future as a non-parent that had been decided. This was a man who had considered having children years before, when he was in a relationship with a woman who had wanted them.

"I didn't do this just for you, you know," he said. "I wouldn't have done it if I didn't want to."

But I already knew that. He isn't, and has never been, a pushover. He does nothing unless he wants to do it. Even so, the thought of someone like him not having a child just didn't feel right, that day.

And sometimes, it still doesn't. Every great now and then, it tears at my soul just a little bit to know that if I wanted a child, he would be all too happy to have one with me.

-

Even when we make the right choice, there's bound to be a little something passed over here or there, so why not indulge every now and then by dipping imaginatively into a parallel life? That I sometimes look at Husband and imagine what our child might look and/or act like doesn't mean I'm second-guessing my choice. That I imagine what it might be like to toss a child into a pile of leaves or tuck one into bed doesn't mean I want that life any more than fantasizing about being a ship captain means I want to quit my job and begin a study of navigation, ocean currents, or the proper names of a ship's parts. It's no more unusual to wonder "what if?" about children than it is to wonder "what if?" about having chosen a different college major.

Refusing to ask questions often means there's some fear about the answers—and that's a pretty compelling reason to ask them, in the first place. The questions are healthy; after all, this is the rest of your life you're talking about.

TEN

TEN KEY POINTS TO REMEMBER

1. It's *your* life.

2. When entering into a relationship, the earlier you talk about children, the better.

3. The more adamantly you insist to your new partner, "I'm not going to change my mind," the better.

4. People say things without thinking. "You'll change your mind" is one of those things. It's automatic. If it's an acquaintance or a stranger at a party who says it, for all of the meaning behind it, they may as well be delivering the small-talk, "I'm fine, and you?" And just as you've grown accustomed to saying, "Oh, fine!" when everything is in the toilet and you want to swim in a tub of gin, you can grow accustomed to saying, "Mm, yep, maybe" when someone says "You'll change your mind." Why bother with a conversation about it with someone who doesn't even know you?

5. On the other hand, if the person insisting you'll change your mind is someone who matters to you, a conversation is more than warranted.

6. Because having children is the obvious choice for the majority of the people, it's just a fact that many of them won't understand why you don't want them, and they'll wonder what you're going to do with your life if you don't have them. If you've seen the second *Sex and the City* movie, you as a child-free person probably have the scene with Carrie and Mr. Big at the wedding reception permanently lodged in your brain. (This was probably the only good scene in that ridiculous movie.)

   If you haven't seen it: Mr. Big and Carrie are greeted by a newly married couple, the female half of which compares herself to Carrie. "I *am* you!" she says. She and her husband then go on to share the wonderful news: they're planning to have a baby. When they ask Carrie when she's having one, Carrie begins (as we've been conditioned to do) by reassuring the couple that she really, truly *loves* children, but they just aren't for her and Big. The woman looks at Carrie and Big with very sad, confused eyes, and she and her husband exchange a look you might expect to see in an oncology wing. People don't *get* it. So, they ask questions. As annoying as that can be, maybe try to understand that some people aren't judgmental, but confused and curious. Even I sometimes wonder "Why?" when I—on rare occasions—meet others who don't want children.

7. Don't assume all parents hate you, judge you, think you're a freak, or think you should have children.

The loudest voices are usually the ones that are the most offensive (which means the voices the child-free tend to "hear" most frequently are in the form of articles or blog entries blasting the child-free); don't let them convince you that all parents (or wannabe parents) are out to get you. Most people I've met who have children firmly believe, "If you don't want them, you shouldn't have them." Live and let live.

8. Likewise, try not to let your frustration with all the questions and assumptions about what you're doing, or should do, with your uterus taint your view of anyone who chooses to have children. There's nothing wrong with having children (as long as you're psychologically fit and can afford it) just like there's nothing wrong with not having children. Live and let live.

9. Once again: There's nothing wrong with not wanting to have children.

10. *Enjoy* your freedom!

ABOUT THE AUTHOR

Sylvia D. Lucas is a writer who is, and will remain, happily child-free. She and her husband live together in a house that has a lawn, but no swing set.

CPSIA information can be obtained at www.ICGtesting.com
Printed in the USA
BVOW011453130112

280518BV00008B/8/P